# SEVEN STAGES

*The Beginner's Guide to Dementia*

# DOUG FRANCIS

ADVISE AUTHOR

COPYRIGHT

# CONTENTS

# ❧ I ❧
# SEVEN STAGES - THE BEGINNER'S GUIDE TO DEMENTIA

# INTRODUCTION

I n 2015 a study was released indicating that over 50 million people had been diagnosed with dementia worldwide. This number was predicted to double every 20 years, reaching 75 million in 2030 and 131.5 million in 2050.

Furthermore, it was estimated that 1 out of 10 people who are above the age of 60 have or will have this condition.

This means that you or someone you know is likely to suffer from the symptoms of dementia in your lifetime, and as a result, this gives us a tremendous incentive to learn and know how to care for people living with dementia.

Although it starts with mild symptoms, it can progress to serious stages that can be hard to manage without a clear understanding of what exactly should be done to reduce its severity.

Unlike other diseases, dementia in itself is not a disease, but it is a term that is used to describe a group of symptoms that commonly occur, which can include but are not necessarily limited to problems in reasoning, communication, learning, and memory.

Dementia is often referred to as neuro-cognitive disorder, and caring for a person that has dementia can pose a series of difficult challenges. Patients who have dementia, especially at later stages, need proper care.

Although, as of this time, there is no official cure for dementia, managing it using a series of heavily researched treatments can help improve the symptoms.

This book offers you valuable information and knowledge about dementia. It delves into the vital areas of causes, types, symptoms, the seven stages, any treatment options that can be applied, foods needed for dementia patients to stay healthy, end of life decisions, and most importantly what to do at the very last stage.

I've written with an awareness that it is a problem that can affect both individuals and families alike on deep and often complex levels.

With the knowledge and advice given in this

book, you will have a good understanding and a firm grasp on knowing exactly what you need to do at each stage of dementia care, especially when things take a turn for the worse.

Who should read this book? This book is a vital tool for those who intend to care for a patient, family member, or loved one who has dementia.

If you have a family member who has late stage dementia, look no further, I've taken great efforts in each chapter of this book to inspire you, offer guidance and demonstrate that with the right knowledge, you can manage symptoms and give your family member the care they deserve.

I hope that you find this book useful and that its contents may be of great help on this journey.

## ❧ 2 ❧

# CAUSES AND TYPES OF
# DEMENTIA

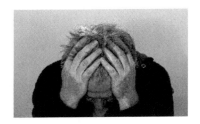

Dementia is a broad term referring to several underlying diseases, and as a result, it presents itself in different ways in different people.

However, in most cases, dementia is associated with the death of brain cells and neurodegenerative diseases.

Interestingly, it is not clear whether brain cell death is what causes dementia, or if it is dementia that leads to the death of brain cells.

But since this is a term that describes many symptoms, other causes may be associated with it.

COMMON CAUSES

Some of the most common causes of dementia include but are not limited to:

## Vascular Disorders

GENERALLY, THESE ARE THE DISORDERS THAT affect the efficient circulation of blood around the whole body.

When one has such conditions, blood circulation in the body and especially in the brain is impaired, leading to the death of brain cells.

Once that happens, memory loss, impaired thinking, and decision making, among other activities, are affected as they are all functions of the brain.

It, therefore, follows that any condition that affects blood circulation is most likely to cause dementia if it is not treated promptly.

## Traumatic Brain Injuries

ACCIDENTS OF A FALLING NATURE, SPECIFICALLY concussions that affect the brain, have been directly linked to dementia. Severe injuries to the brain are a common cause.

Tragically, when the brain is injured, its normal functions are affected, and the chances are that if the necessary treatments are not carried out, the person affected is more likely to suffer from dementia as time progresses.

## Neurological Diseases

MOST NEUROLOGICAL DISORDERS THAT CAUSE degeneration of brain cells have also been found to be among the leading causes of dementia.

Some of these diseases include Alzheimer's disease, Huntington's disease, and Parkinson's disease.

Also, other conditions, such as multiple sclerosis, are said to cause dementia. Most of these diseases are difficult to treat; hence they get worse with time leading to dementia.

# Diseases that Affect the Central Nervous System

DISEASES THAT CAUSE INFECTIONS TO THE CENTRAL nervous system are also among the leading causes of dementia. The two leading diseases in this area are HIV and meningitis.

Their effects over time cause the death of brain cells and the weakening of the body's immune system.

The final effect is, therefore, serious memory loss, an inability to learn, and even difficulties in communication. All these are symptoms of dementia, and hence, these diseases are listed as being known as possible causes.

## Alcohol and Drug Abuse

PROLONGED USE OF ALCOHOL AND OTHER DRUGS that affect the normal functioning of the brain can also lead to dementia.

Although it takes time to manifest, excessive use of alcohol, as well as uncontrolled use of drugs, can eventually lead to brain damage resulting in dementia.

It is thus vital to take or consume alcohol and

drugs in controlled amounts up to the recommended daily limits.

## Build Up of Fluid in the Brain

SOME DISORDERS, SUCH AS SOME TYPES OF hydrocephalus, can lead to a build-up of fluid in the brain. If not treated early enough, such disorders can lead to brain damage, and eventually cause dementia.

Also, brain tumors or growths in the brain can affect its normal functioning, and a resultant severe condition can be dementia.

## Stroke

STROKE AFFECTS ARTERIES AND OTHER BLOOD vessels leading to the brain. As a result, it also affects the supply of oxygen and vital nutrients to the brain.

When a stroke occurs, the normal functioning of the brain is affected, and in some cases, this can result in dementia, or, in more extreme circumstances, death.

Stroke is considered to be one of the leading causes of disability and deaths worldwide.

## TYPES OF DEMENTIA

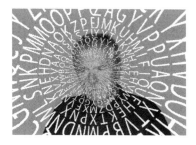

While there are many types of dementia, they can be classified into three groups. This classification is based on the two parts of the brain that are often affected by the condition. In instances where both parts of the brain are affected, one suffers from a mixed type.

Based on this, here are the most common types of dementia:

## **Cortical Dementia**

AS THE NAME SUGGESTS, THESE ARE DEMENTIA TYPES that affect the cerebral cortex or simply the brain's outer layer. This part of the brain is responsible for communication as well as memory.

Any disease that, affects this part of the brain results in loss of memory and the inability to understand language. The most common forms as well as causes of cortical dementia are:

- Creutzfeldt-Jacob disease
- Alzheimer's disease

## Sub-Cortical Dementia

Just as was the case with the first type, the name of this type of dementia suggests that it affects the part of the brain that is beneath the cortex. This part of the brain is responsible for activity and thinking.

Therefore, anyone suffering from a condition that affects this part of the brain is more likely to have problems related to decision-making and the ability to start activities.

However, such people do not have any challenges related to language or being forgetful, as is the case with the first type of dementia.

Diseases that cause this type of dementia include:

- Huntington's disease
- HIV
- Parkinson's disease

## Mixed Dementia

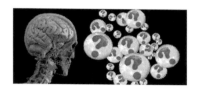

Unlike the other two types already described, this type tends to be more severe. It affects both parts of the brain resulting in paralysis.

It happens when cortical and subcortical dementias occur simultaneously. What this means is that the patient suffers from symptoms associated with the above two types together.

It is, therefore, the worst type of dementia, and it often leads to death quickly. The most commonly diagnosed form of this type of dementia is when both Alzheimer's disease and vascular dementia occur together.

It is worth noting that the examples of diseases cited here are only the most common ones that are associated with dementia. Others are also responsible for the above types of dementia, although they are more rarely reported.

The most commonly reported diseases often

referred to as dementia may include Down Syndrome, Normal Pressure Hydrocephalus, Frontotemporal Dementia, and or Posterior Cortical Atrophy. All of these diseases can also lead to symptoms of dementia.

It goes without saying that if they are diagnosed early, they can result in a much higher quality of care being delivered as consideration is applied, and techniques can be used to mitigate symptoms, resulting in a better quality of life for the patient.

# COMMON SYMPTOMS OF DEMENTIA

A person with dementia will often show many symptoms that demonstrate the severity as well as the type.

However, as already said, dementia in itself is not a disease but rather a combination of different illnesses.

Besides, some symptoms can easily manifest themselves and are easy to tell that the underlying condition is dementia.

On the other hand, certain symptoms can only be identified by caregivers or health professionals.

## COMMON SYMPTOMS

### Mood Changes

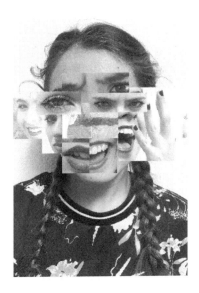

People with dementia often experience sudden and unexplained changes in their moods. They often start as minor or daily mood changes before they transform into more serious mood swings at a later stage.

Although some people take them as normal, the fact is that if they are prolonged, they are an indication of a serious underlying condition.

## Personality Changes

WHEN AN AGING OR ELDERLY PERSON SUDDENLY gets fearful, suspicious, or becomes easily irritated by petty issues, there is reason to believe it may be a result of dementia.

At the late stage, the symptoms described above tend to get more serious, and the person displaying this behavior may become increasingly difficult for caregivers to deal with.

## Memory Loss

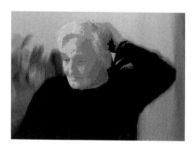

AS ILLUSTRATED IN THE TYPES OF DEMENTIA, THERE are certain causes of this condition that affect the cortical part of the brain responsible for memory.

As a result, it is common for people with this type of dementia to lose memory. The loss is often evidenced by such people asking the same question over and over.

If that happens to be observed repeatedly, there is a high probability that the person may have dementia.

## Less Interest in Taking Initiatives

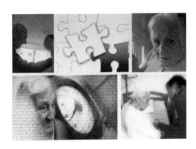

A PERSON WITH DEMENTIA CAN LACK SIGNS OF ambition and may constantly seem unwilling to take initiative or start new projects.

If you ask them to accompany you somewhere or start a project with you, it is also likely they will be unable to comply or take it seriously.

If you notice this behavior in a friend or family member, and it is becoming a repeated pattern that is out of the ordinary, it is a good time to start suspecting dementia and begin to follow best practices to mitigate this behavior.

### Difficulty in Completing Normal Tasks

If it suddenly becomes difficult for one to do normal chores at home, then that too can be a sign of dementia. It can start with tough tasks and may later progress to much simpler ones. It is not uncommon for someone with dementia to be unable to have difficulty doing things we take for granted, for example, cooking a simple meal or preparing drinks. Tasks that you would find incredibly easy and would only take a few minutes to accomplish.

### Communication Problems

With dementia, simple words often become complex, and people suffering from the condition forget simple words. That implies that communication becomes a great challenge as language and communicating effectively can become a real problem for people who have dementia.

### Misplacing and Forgetting Things

Forgetting where one placed everyday items such as keys, phone, and wallet is also a sign of dementia. Patients with this condition can easily forget where they placed their items on a daily basis. They should thus be helped in locating them, especially when it becomes a common occurrence.

Other symptoms of dementia also manifest depending on the underlying conditions of the patient. The above-discussed symptoms are, however, the most common ones. They easily manifest, and as one grows older, they tend to worsen.

❧ 4 ❧

# THE SEVEN STAGES OF
# DEMENTIA

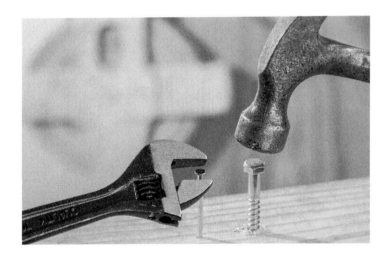

D ementia is a disease that has been
thoroughly researched by numerous
medical professionals and subject matter
experts.

It has been determined that the disease referred

to as dementia is often categorized into seven unique stages:

## STAGE ONE: NO SIGNS OF IMPAIRMENT

At this initial stage, the patient does not show any signs of memory impairment. The condition has just started and is undetectable.

It is also referred to as the 'no cognitive decline stage' without any symptoms at all.

## STAGE TWO: VERY MILD COGNITIVE DECLINE

The patient starts to experience typical forgetfulness. Since there are no obvious signs of any serious underlying condition, it looks like normal aging symptoms.

Common mistakes include small misplacements that family members and even a physician may not notice unless under serious scrutiny.

## STAGE THREE: MILD COGNITIVE IMPAIRMENT

This stage of dementia is often characterized by mild symptoms such as general forgetfulness and minor communication problems.

If it is diagnosed early and treated almost immediately, it can be mitigated significantly.

## STAGE FOUR: MILD DEMENTIA

At this stage, cognitive impairment becomes much more easily observed. One experiences memory problems, language issues, decision-making, and other problems associated with the disease.

At this stage, problems begin to affect normal daily routines. It is evidenced by symptoms that include difficulty in completing normal everyday tasks, confusion, and personality changes.

## STAGE FIVE: MODERATE DEMENTIA

At this stage, the person affected needs help since their daily routine becomes a challenge. Everyday tasks such as getting dressed, combing hair, preparing food, have all become almost impossible.

The patient also may experience sleep disorders, changes in personality, and be easily disturbed by things that other people tend more often than not to simply brush off.

More care is, therefore, preferred to help manage the condition as it moves into a category commonly described as 'late stage dementia'.

## STAGE SIX: SEVERE COGNITIVE DECLINE

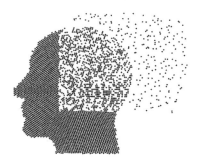

Loss of memory, an inability to communicate, difficulty in eating, and inability to control the bladder are the symptoms experienced at this stage of the disease.

What this implies for caregivers is that complete and full-time care is a must for patients suffering from this severe stage of dementia. Even at night, such patients need care since they also tend to have sleeping problems.

## STAGE SEVEN: VERY SEVERE COGNITIVE IMPAIRMENT / UNCONSCIOUSNESS

The patient's health at this stage has deteriorated completely, such that even sitting and holding one's head up is impossible. Intensive care is, therefore, needed to sustain one's life.

The patient has difficulty staying warm as their body often tends to be cold, and more often than not, the patient remains in a state of unconsciousness.

In the final stage of dementia, it may be hard to interact or make any sort of meaningful connection, but it is also the point at which this person will need your love the most.

It is a time in which we must bravely accept the inevitable and make final arrangements for the impending death of our loved one.

# USEFUL TREATMENTS FOR
## DEMENTIA

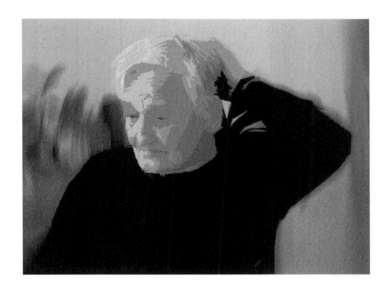

lthough the death of brain cells cannot be reversed, there are a couple of treatments that can help reduce the severity of the condition.

It is also worth noting that if dementia is a result of treatable serious underlying causes, it may be possible to manage it.

The first stage to managing the disease is, therefore, to understand the underlying cause so that appropriate measures can be taken in advance.

In the US, for instance, there are a couple of medications that have been approved for use in the management of the symptoms of Alzheimer's disease, one of the leading causes of dementia.

The drugs include Galantamine (Reminyl), Donepezil (Aricept), and Tacrine (Cognex). It is important to note that these drugs should be used with caution and under guidance of a highly trained physician.

## ❦ 6 ❧
## FOOD AND NUTRITION SUPPORTING LATE STAGE DEMENTIA

During late stage dementia, many patients often lose interest in food.

For instance, they tend to skip important mealtimes, and even when they eat, they still do not eat as much as they did before.

The resultant effect of such a habit is that the patient may lack vital vitamins and minerals that are necessary for maintaining optimum health.

Such people need support since skipping meals or failing to get vital nutrients only accelerates the degeneration of their bodies.

In this section of this book, I can offer a few useful tips regarding foods needed to cope with late stage dementia.

## CONSUMPTION AND NUTRITION RECOMMENDATIONS

### Find a Quiet Eating Place

People with dementia are not comfortable eating in noisy places. Therefore, before we look at what is good for them to eat, the first thing to do is to make sure that the environment around them is quiet.

That means that you need to switch off the radio, CD player, and even the TV.

Any form of noise from any source easily disturbs them, and it also affects their eating habits. So, make sure that they are not disrupted as you feed them.

### Serve Meals at Regular Times of the Day

MEALS FOR PEOPLE WHO HAVE DEMENTIA SHOULD BE served at the same time each day.

Any changes, even if small, can greatly affect their eating habits. They may fail to take meals served at unusual times. It is thus great to create consistency regarding mealtimes.

Most importantly, ensure that as the person in

charge of providing care for them, your patients do not miss a single meal.

Missing meals only serves to aggravate the problem and results in reduced hunger and stomach issues when food is consumed irregularly.

## Use Colorful Plates

DEMENTIA INTERFERES WITH VITAL PARTS OF THE brain, and in its late stage, the condition makes it hard for patients to recognize food served to them.

It is, therefore, advisable that you use colorful plates or other utensils that are quite easily recognized by the patient.

Using such items makes it easy for them to see and realize that it is time to take their food.

In some instances, you may need to spoon-feed them if they cannot consume their meals alone.

## Offer One Food at a Time

INSTEAD OF FILLING THE PLATE WITH LOTS OF different food, it is advisable that you simply offer one food at a time if you want your patient to eat contentedly.

Remember that anything that creates confusion or adds too much information at once in a short space of time is more likely to affect their eating habits.

## Ensure that Dentures are Tight-Fitting

IF YOUR PATIENT HAS DENTURES, MAKE SURE THAT they are tight-fitting. They can easily cause problems such as choking while they are eating.

If the dentures do not fit properly, it may be advisable that you resort to soft foods that don't require chewing, so simply take them out for the patient and make efforts to find them a pair of dentures that fit well.

## Recommended Types of Foods

DUE TO THEIR SEVERE HEALTH CONDITION, patients who have dementia should only be fed specific types of food.

Such food should supply the needed nutrients and also be easy for them to swallow without any problem.

· · ·

***Here are the foods that come highly recommended for patients with Dementia:***

• HIGH-CALORIE HEALTHY FOODS LIKE PROTEIN milkshakes

• FINGER FOODS LIKE SMALL SANDWICHES, FRESH fruits, vegetables and cheese

• MULTIVITAMIN TABLETS, POWDER, CAPSULES, AND liquids

ALSO, WHEN IT COMES TO COOKING FOOD FOR people with this condition, it is recommended that you use healthy fats such as olive oil.

If you are concerned about calorie intake, you can use butter, mayonnaise, and extra cooking oil when preparing the food.

However, if the patient has some other chronic illnesses such as diabetes, you may have to consult a doctor first on the right oils to use.

## Dealing With Food Swallowing Problems

AS DEMENTIA PROGRESSES TO THE VERY LATE STAGE, chewing and swallowing become a real problem for patients. Without proper care, such problems can reduce their lifespan, yet they would live longer if they received proper care.

It is important to note that swallowing problems can also lead to serious issues such as pneumonia. Such a disease for an already ailing patient can only cause increased hardship.

It is, therefore, good to discuss a few ways of dealing with the common problem of dementia patients being unable to swallow.

One way to solve the swallowing problem is by grinding food or liquefying it just as you would for a baby. Also, make sure that food is cut into smaller pieces that are soft and easy to eat.

That way, you reduce the chance of your patient choking on their food. It is a highly recommended method, and it works great, especially during the last stage of dementia.

Soft foods, such as milkshakes, ice cream, gelatin, yogurt, and soups, should be served often as they are easy to swallow.

Try to make sure the person caring for the patient is always offering food of this nature—any other types of food risk causing swallowing problems that put the life of the patient at risk.

Serving slightly warm or cold drinks is also another way to deal with swallowing problems among patients with dementia.

Research has shown that cold drinks are easier to swallow compared to those that are hot. So, if you want to offer a drink to your patient who has dementia, make sure that it is a cold drink.

A few more things to keep in mind include prohibiting the use of straws, avoiding situations where the caregiver is forced to hurry the patient in eating their meals, or feeding a patient when they are lying down.

Make sure that you put the patient in an upright sitting position for at least twenty minutes before and after their meals.

# ❧ 7 ❧

## END OF LIFE DECISIONS

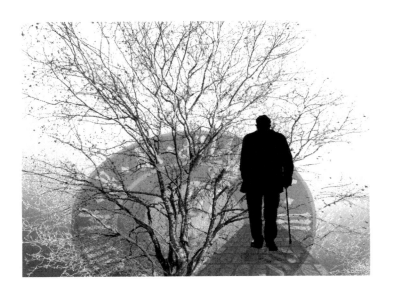

End of life decisions are also part of caregiving for patients with dementia. Essentially, when the diagnosis is made, and there is evidence that the underlying condition is incurable, plans should be made for the end of life.

This requirement, however, differs from one person to another. It is, however, recommended that any important decisions should be made when the patient still knows what is happening and can make informed decisions.

In circumstances where important decisions are not made early enough, the end of life decisions for a patient with late stage dementia become a bit complicated.

Nevertheless, it is still important to make sure that everything possible is done to give the patient the best environment even when their condition seems to not get any better with time.

Provided they can still speak, they should be helped to make vital decisions so that problems do not arise later, especially when they die, and there are no wills or decisions made.

## How and Why End of Life Decisions are Vital

First, quality of life is very vital, and the patient should be assisted in making important healthcare decisions that they want. Leaving them without a healthcare plan amounts to negligence, and they may suffer a lot.

For instance, they should be helped to choose medicines that can help manage to delay the symptoms of the disease affecting them.

It is, however, good to note that some patients may not want such care. It is thus great to explain to them if they can understand that having such a plan is for their benefit.

If the patient's condition is already worse, and they cannot make any decision, then someone else close to them can help make them.

Preferably, this is a family member or anyone that understands the patient's behavior or what they liked while they were healthy.

The person can then help in making treatment decisions and goals for the remaining period.

More specifically, the person making the decisions should weigh the pros and cons of each plan, and pick one that is most likely to help manage or improve the patient's condition.

With dementia, end of life decisions make it simpler for caregivers to face the tough situation that awaits them as days move on towards the very severe end-stage.

But even at such a stage when hope is no more, care should still be provided.

It is still vital and should be one of the goals of anyone affected by a person's condition, whether they are family members of just close friends concerned with the health of their peers.

## Important Questions to Ask about End of Life Decisions

TO GET THE BEST CARE OR MEDICAL OPTION FOR your beloved person who has dementia, it would be great to pose a few questions.

The aim of doing so is to weigh options carefully before a decision on which route is the best among the available alternatives is then made.

*HERE ARE A COUPLE OF IMPORTANT QUESTIONS to ask:*

1. IS HOME HOSPICE THE BEST OPTION, OR SHOULD you take him/her to a care center away from home?

. . .

2. IF HOME HOSPICE IS PREFERRED, ARE THERE necessary facilities needed to support their life, especially during the last severe stage?

3. HOW WILL THE PATIENT'S CONDITION AFFECT the rest of the family?

4. WILL THEIR CONDITION BRING EVERYTHING TO A standstill and cause more problems?

5. WHAT IS THE BEST WAY TO PROMOTE THE wellbeing of the patient and offer them comfort, even when they can no longer notice the difference?

6. WHAT ARE THE WORST EXPECTED SITUATIONS towards the end of life?

7. IS THERE A GOOD DOCTOR OR CAREGIVER WHO can help handle the situation near you?

. . .

8. IF NOT, WHAT PLANS ARE THERE TO GET ONE who has the experience in handling such life-changing situations?

PROVIDED YOU HAVE A PATIENT OR PERSON suffering from late-stage dementia at home, you may want to ask these questions.

They are, however, not meant to complicate things but to help you choose the best package that can make things easier for the patient.

If you have never faced such a situation or seen anyone at such a stage, you need to prepare. Things can get worse towards the end.

It is, therefore, very vital to prepare well and be ready to face any difficulties that come with this stage.

## Depression and How to Avoid It

FAMILY CAREGIVERS OFTEN HAVE TO SACRIFICE A lot to take care of persons with dementia.

Doing so, especially towards the last stage, can be so demanding. It is also a stressful situation that begs for full-time care.

One may even have to leave work completely to

provide care. Such caregiving responsibilities can sometimes lead to depression.

Problems with depression can get worse than the normal stressful situation, especially if the person giving care is doing it alone or with little support. That means that one will be fighting two problems at once.

In such moments, the depressed caregiver will start looking forward to the day when the patient will die to provide relief.

Indeed, it is the worst situation one can ever face. It is thus vital to understand it and find ways of reducing the chances of getting depression.

To avoid depression, there is a need to share responsibilities and let the burden of providing care be shared among many.

Counseling services are also vital to help give hope to the stressed family members and especially caregivers.

That's the best way to manage fatigue, hardships, and daily sacrifices that come with having a person with late stage dementia.

## THE VERY LAST STAGE

The very end-stage of dementia refers to the last few months, weeks, and days when the patient's condition worsens. At this phase, it can neither be reversed nor managed anymore.

This is the stage where the caregiver sees the real signs of dying, and no remedial measures or treatments seem to help contain the situation.

As a family caregiver, this stage requires real courage and readiness to face the situation.

It is, therefore, vital to realize when this phase starts so that the right actions and decisions can be made.

Towards the last few months, a couple of things will happen that, if monitored well, indicate that the patient is going towards the end of life.

## *Most of the common symptoms at this stage include:*

• INCREASED VISITS TO THE HOSPITAL

• A FRESH DIAGNOSIS OF A TERMINAL DISEASE SUCH as heart failure and cancer

• CONTINUED DETERIORATION IN HEALTH OR minimal response to treatment

## The Last Few Weeks

WHEN A FEW WEEKS ARE LEFT, THE PATIENT'S condition continues to deteriorate, and numerous signs could be suggesting that only a few weeks are left.

*IN MOST CASES, THE PATIENT WILL SHOW THE following serious signs:*

. . .

- SHALLOW AND SOMETIMES DIFFICULT BREATHS

- INABILITY TO SWALLOW FOOD

- RESTLESSNESS AND TERMINAL AGITATION

## Final Days

THE FINAL DAYS ARE OFTEN MARKED WITH GREATER difficulty and severity of the condition.

*MORE SPECIFICALLY, THE PATIENT EXPERIENCES a couple of signs that include:*

- LEGS, HANDS, AND BODY INCREASINGLY BECOMING cold

- SLOW DRIFT INTO UNCONSCIOUSNESS

## What You Can Do at the Very Last Stage

ALTHOUGH THERE IS LITTLE THAT CAN BE DONE TO help the patient at this stage, your loving presence is still valuable and important for them.

You shouldn't leave them alone even when they are already unconscious of what is happening.

There are a couple of things you can do that will demonstrate your love for them. They may not see it, but the fact is that they will feel it even at their death bed.

Some of the things that you can do in the final weeks and days to support them are generally the simple yet vital acts of love. You can, for instance, hold their hands, play some cool low-tone music or simply sit with them.

At all costs, you should never leave them or simply sit waiting for their final moment.

Also, if the patient is experiencing a lot of pain, you should talk to a physician on the possibility of palliative care during the last days.

Another great gift and demonstration of love that you can show to the patient during their last stages is ensuring that all their things are in order.

All financial, as well as healthcare preparations and any claims, should be made ready with your attorney.

Also, you should make sure that there will be no crisis once they are no more.

It thus makes sense to have all arrangements set in readiness to meet all hard circumstances in the last days.

## A Peaceful Transition

FINALLY, IT IS YOUR RESPONSIBILITY AS THE FAMILY caregiver to ensure that the dementia patient makes their final transition in peace.

One way to do so is to avoid any activities that can lead them to death before it reaches their final day.

Help them manage pain through care and presence. Most importantly, keep them comfortable to the very last minute.

Caring for an individual in the family with dementia is not only challenging, but it can also be extremely stressful.

The situation can even cause depression for those involved in providing care, especially when support is provided at home.

Indeed, without a proper guide on what to do, especially in the last stages, things can get extremely confusing and scary.

However, with the knowledge of what one should expect at such stages, things can be made simple through proper planning at every stage.

The most important thing to note is that dementia is not a disease with a cure.

Instead, it is a term that describes a couple of

underlying terminal diseases that are often difficult to treat or manage.

Helping patients with dementia is one of the greatest things a person can do for them when their life changes completely.

As discussed in this book, a time comes when they are unable to move their bodies, swallow, sit, or sleep comfortably alone.

Being there to help them in such circumstances is an absolute blessing. However, handling their situation without knowing exactly what should be done at each stage can be a challenge.

Things can only be easy when you know what to do as a caregiver. Remember that even decision-making and communication often becomes challenging for such patients.

This book was intended to help people who have patients at home suffering from dementia.

Although it targeted those with last stage dementia, even those with patients at the very initial stages will still find this resource useful in their daily care routine. Indeed, there is a lot to learn about dementia.

The most important areas, as shown in this book include symptoms, the right foods, end of life decisions, and, most importantly, what to do as the patient enters the very last stage of dementia and despair begins to set in.

As we come to the end of this book, I hope it has helped you understand all aspects of dementia and has better prepared you to take care of a family member or loved one.

The best way to master this material is to read again and again or simply refer to it when the need arises.

Thank you for taking the time to educate yourself on this topic further, and I wish you and your family my heartfelt condolences as you embark on this difficult journey of caring for a loved one.

SINCERELY,

Doug Francis

## ABOUT THE AUTHOR

Doug Francis is a subject matter expert on health, fitness and nutrition topics. He is a passionate author of high quality titles offering practical information and advice for his readers.

**Wait, before you go...**

I really can't thank you enough for taking the time to read "Seven Stages." I know this topic can be hard for many to deal with.

It is of great importance to me that this book is the best it can possibly be and your feedback means the world to me. I read every single review and take feedback seriously in an effort to improve this book.

Thank you so much for your support!

Sincerely,
Doug Francis

**Leave a Review on Amazon.com**

https://www.amazon.com/review/create-review?
asin=%B0879GZ2CL

# REFERENCES

Branger, C., Burton, R., O'Connell, M. E., Stewart, N., & Morgan, D. (2016). Coping with cognitive impairment and dementia: Rural caregivers' perspectives. *Dementia*, *15*(4), 814-831.

Brooker, D. (2003). What is person-centered care in dementia?. *Reviews in clinical gerontology*, *13*(3), 215-222.

Engdahl, S. (2013). *Dementia*. Greenhaven Publishing LLC.

Kovach, C.R. (1997). *Late-Stage Dementia: A Basic Guide*. Taylor & Francis.

# ADVISE AUTHOR PUBLISHING

Please take a moment to review some of the other amazing titles associated with Advise Author Publishing now available in the Amazon Kindle store:

**1.)** The Beginner's Guide to Blogging: 25 Essential Tips For Turning Your Blogging Passion Into Profits

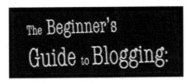

## The Beginner's Guide to Blogging:

## 25 Essential Tips for Turning your Blogging Passion into Profit$

### David Grete

**Have you noticed how some bloggers make six or seven-figure incomes while others struggle to even make $100?** What if I could teach you some key skills and habits that could make your blog a true success financially?

One of the biggest secrets I can share about blogging, one that I quickly came to understand from other successful communicators, is that you have to be **passionate** about what you're writing. But this book has so much more to offer.

**In this book, you'll find easy step-by-step instructions on how to:**

* Setup your very own blog.

* Analyze and select a specific niche that is both profitable and that you are passionate about.

* Promote and market your blog using several proven social media marketing strategies.

* Apply basic content strategy and design elements to your blog posts to make them go viral.

* Apply 25 essential blogging tips that can help you turn passion into profit.

*While you may not get instantly rich from blogging it is something you can easily build upon in your spare time and expand into a full-fledged career path. In this book you will learn everything you need to know to get a huge advantage in blogging by standing on the shoulders of some of the most successful bloggers ever to put words on a page.*

For less than a cup of coffee, this book will literally teach you how to turn your passion into profit, become your own boss and eventually leave the day job behind!

The Beginner's
Guide to Blogging:

**25** Essential Tips
for **Turning**
your Blogging
**Passion** into
**Profit$** [DG]

David Grete

**2.)** She Gets It Done: How Successful Women Manage Their Time

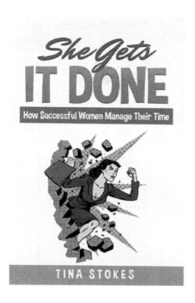

In **She Gets It Done™** you will learn:

✓ How to transform yourself into an extremely productive person.

✓ Tips and tricks that will show you how to work smarter, not harder.

✓ How to free up massive amounts of time by looking at the big picture and delegating tasks.

✓ How to organize your time in a more logical and efficient way, leaving more time for you.

✓ How to prioritize your most important tasks and eliminate wasted time on the things that simply don't matter much.

Do you think it's impossible to find the time to do things that make you happy? Think again because, I've done it and now I want to show you how!

There's no time to wait. The clock is ticking and we need to make the most of it. Grab a copy of this book and let me show you how to really make the most from your time!

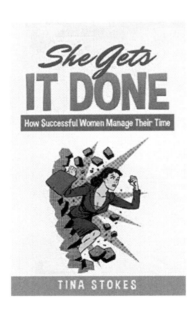

**3.) Herbal Medicine for Everyone: The Begin-**

ner's Guide to Healing Common Illnesses with 20 Medicinal Herbs

**Herbal Medicine for Everyone™ is the go to guide for alleviating common illnesses through the use of over 20 medicinal herbs.**

*The number of handbooks and guides covering this topic can make finding the right book extremely overwhelming.*

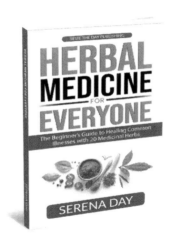

✓ Fortunately, it doesn't take a genius to begin harnessing the power of herbal medicine to cure common illnesses, it only takes some basic training and initiative.

Herbal Medicine for Everyone highlights effective herbs and homemade remedies that assist in the body's natural ability to fight off infections and ultimately cure itself of the common illnesses that plague us frequently.

This book will transform readers into junior herbalists who can easily recognize the most abundant and effective medicinal herbs that they can use to craft powerful remedies for common illnesses.

★ **Included are remedies proven to be effective in reducing the severity of headaches, fevers, allergies and many other common ailments. Junior herbalists will learn the essential knowledge they need to transform into highly skilled naturopathic caregivers and gain a unique ability to apply herbal medicine effectively.**

**Herbal Medicine for Everyone teaches you how to use herbs as preventative and restorative medicine with:**

✓ An Herbal Medicine Orientation provides the building blocks of knowledge when it comes to purchasing, making, and using herbal medicine in an effective manner.

✓ An Overview of Popular Herbs teaches you how to select the appropriate herbs for your medicinal herbal pantry.

✓ 20+ Herbal Remedies for Common Ailments with step-by-step instructions on how to make them in the comfort of your own home.

*You'll learn how to alleviate stress with linden, soothe and comfort burns using marshmallow and detoxify your body using dandelion.*

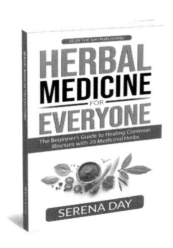

Get a copy of "Herbal Medicine for Everyone" today and ditch the store bought meds forever.

## 4.) Seven Stages: The Beginner's Guide to Dementia

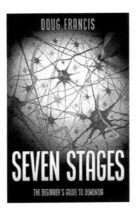

*It is very hard watching a loved one suffer. When taking care of a loved one there is no doubt that the late-stage crisis that comes with dementia can be extremely hard to manage and cope with.*

Although the condition strikes differently and in its own way depending on the individual, there is a real need for guidance when it comes to proper care for patients and loved ones.

It is even more important if you intend to become a caregiver to an elderly father or mother suffering from this condition. *Helping people to more confidently take care of a friend or family member during this difficult time was what inspired me to write "Seven Stages: The Beginner's Guide to Dementia."*

Statistics show that the likelihood of one suffering from dementia increases with age, and it is extremely common in those of sixty yearss of age and older. This book was written with a few important goals in mind.

### In this book you will learn:

✓ *The many causes and types of dementia.*

✓ *Common symptoms and an overview of the seven stages of dementia.*

✓ *Well researched nutritional guidelines to help prepare healthy meals that can assist in mitigating the symptoms of dementia.*

✓ *Difficult end of life decisions that may need to be made for patients suffering late stage dementia.*

✓ *Taking care of someone that is in the very last stage of dementia.*

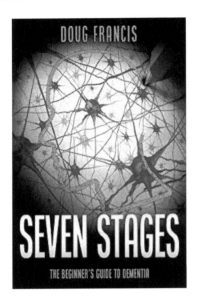